NATURE'S CHILD

HEALING CHILDREN FROM THE INSIDE OUT

PAULA J JOHNSON, ND, OTR

BALBOA.
PRESS

A DIVISION OF HAY HOUSE

Balboa Press books may be ordered through booksellers or by contacting:

Balboa Press
A Division of Hay House
1663 Liberty Drive
Bloomington, IN 47403
www.balboapress.com
1 (877) 407-4847

Print information available on the last page.

ISBN: 978-1-5043-7843-7 (sc)
ISBN: 978-1-5043-7844-4 (hc)
ISBN: 978-1-5043-7860-4 (e)

Library of Congress Control Number: 2017905457

Balboa Press rev. date: 07/19/2017

CONTENTS

ACKNOWLEDGMENTS

When I first started writing this book, I had no idea how it would change me as a person. The process of finding my voice to a subject that I'm so deeply passionate about has been such a gift. There have been so many instrumental people who have encouraged me, inspired me, and helped me along the way.

To my inspiring teachers at the Naturopathic Institute of Therapies and Education and Trinity College of Natural Health, thank you for opening my eyes to Naturopathy, it's miracles and for providing a sense of "Hope" to any health issue.

To my colleagues, Crystal M, Laura A, Dr. Kribs, and the South Team, who taught me so much and supported me throughout this process.

To Judy B, and Ashley P, thank you for making sense out of my long, run on paragraphs, you're truly amazing, patient, and kind.

To my loving mother, who inspired all of us by your example of living healthy.

To my loving family of crazy health nuts, and especially my brother Chris, thank you for all your knowledge and encouragement to keep moving forward.

To all my friends who encouraged me and believed in me from the start, especially girls group, you all kept me going.

To my soul sisters Stacy, Celine, and Molly, thank you for being there my entire life!

To my children, Mack, Hayley & Natalie, thank you for teaching me what children really need – space to be who they are.

To Dave, whose love encouraged me to believe in myself. Your firm push kept me going. I Love You & Thank You!

Lastly, I want to thank the many children and families over the years who because you let me in your home and hearts, I was inspired to write this book. You were my reason to see a whole new way to raise children to live a happy, healthy life.

INTRODUCTION

What has happened to our children? Have you noticed that children don't seem as resilient and healthy as they used to be? When looking at the amount of children in the United States that have a diagnosis of ADHD, autism, allergies or any of the other many childhood illnesses, the question "Why so many children?" comes to mind. The amount of prescription drugs has dramatically increased in the past 10 years, with one in five children on at least one drug for asthma, ADHD, along with being over prescribed antibiotics. In 2008, 2.8 million children between the ages of six and twelve were prescribed stimulant medications for ADHD Why? Are we missing the big picture? Is it not all about treating symptoms, but rather looking at what is really causing our children to be so sick, hyperactive, and "bouncing off the walls?"

I have always had a passion for children and health and have worked for over 30 years as a pediatric Occupational Therapist. My job involves helping families to help their children with such skills as feeding, using their hands to play with toys, move their bodies to explore the world, along with helping them to interpret sensations they receive from their senses such as smell, taste, sight, sound, touch, movement, and the position of their body. During the past 20 years,

I have been working with young children, ages birth to age 3, for an early intervention program called Early On. This is a home based program where I work with the family in their home so they can help their children learn a variety of skills. Many of the children have developmental delays or an established condition such as prematurity that makes them at risk for having developmental concerns. Over the past 15 years, I started to notice that these children were becoming so much more ill than the children before them and I started to question why these children appeared more immune compromised. I also noticed that my approach to working with these children was changing and that the sensory techniques I had used in the past to help children with self regulation and calming their nervous system wasn't working anymore either. As an Occupational Therapist (OT), it is common to work with children with sensory processing disorders where touch, movement, sound and other sensory stimulation can either be painful or they seek stimulation way more than others. Sensory strategies such as deep pressure touch, and engaging in pushing, pulling or moving heavy objects which OT's call "heavy work" didn't have the same calming effect which lead me to question if something more organic was going on.

So why are the sensory strategies to help children calm down that were so successful 15 years ago not working anymore today? There has to be something more going on. Is there something in the water? Could it be something they're eating? My quest began to find the answers and I started taking any class I could find that talked about how food could impact behavior. It was then that I found a class that talked about the connection between food, specifically proteins that are in wheat products (gluten) and dairy products (casein) and how these undigested proteins impacted children who had weak digestion, such as children with autism. This was fascinating and I had to share it with my families that had children with autism. These families were as fascinated as I was and they began slowing taking out specific foods and to their surprise and mine, these children improved. I was blown away! These children were changing so quickly and were improving in such ways as better eye contact, sleeping through the night, improved attention, less tantrums, and some started to say their first words. I had no clue why this was working, but all I knew was when these kids did not drink milk or eat bread products, they improved. Wow, this was fascinating! That's when I knew FOOD is powerful!

What else was in food that could either harm or help the brain of children or adults for that matter? I began researching how natural strategies such as food, herbs, essential oils, and other natural remedies helped these kids far better than medication. What started as an interest in finding more ways to help these children with sensory needs, ended up eight years later with a degree as a Naturopathic Doctor or "Naturopath."

For the past eight years, I have combined my knowledge as an OT with my knowledge as a Naturopath and found natural ways to help children with a variety of health issues. It is amazing how we don't even question how our skin heals up when we get scratched. So why would it be any different for ear infections or allergies? The body wants to heal itself and has this innate intelligence to do so. Masking symptoms with medications does not take care of the problem, but only covers up what originally caused the problem in the first place. As a Naturopath, the focus is to bring the body back in balance and look at what caused the problem rather than just trying to get rid of symptoms. Naturopaths are not medical doctors and, therefore, do not **treat, cure, diagnose**, or **prescribe**, but rather educate and empower.

There are so many simple, easy, and practical ways for families to naturally help their children without always having to medicate them. This is why it's important to see your medical doctor for annual check-ups and a Naturopath for prevention strategies for overall health.

My intention for writing this book is to help families understand reasons why the body becomes ill in the first place, how to prevent from getting ill, and then provide a simple guide of different ways to help bring the body back in balance so that healing takes place naturally, as nature intended.

PART ONE

CHAPTER 1

Good Health is Natural

Health is a natural part of life. The body was created perfectly and has an innate intelligence to stay in balance, working very hard every second to do so. We function best when there is a balance of proper foods, exercise, and serenity. A perfect example of this is the people who live in the "blue zones" of the world, which are areas where people live the longest and are the healthiest. These people live to be well over the age of 100, are the farthest from health care, have no symptoms, and live in underdeveloped areas. These people live in harmony with each other, the environment, and enjoy life and their good health.

So why in the richest and most developed country in the world do we focus on illness and disease rather than wellness? Last year we spent 3.8 trillion dollars on health care alone. Obviously, there is a health crisis, but why? It has become common to talk about our symptoms and compare who has more symptoms and who is worse off. We focus on the disease and manage it through the use of drugs and surgery in order to "fix" the body. When we relieve symptoms by taking medications or performing surgery to remove something, we are often only compounding the problem rather than looking at what caused the problem to begin with. Wellness focuses on keeping the body in balance so that the "cause" of the problem does not get to the point where symptoms appear.

Your Body Is Always Talking

Our body has an innate intelligence and will do anything to survive. One of the laws of the universe is "cause and effect." Our body, too, follows this law and will respond accordingly to whatever happens to it. In natural health, there is a law about how the body heals itself, which is called the "Herrings Law of Cure." This law states that the body heals from the inside out, top down, and in the reverse order that symptoms occur. What? Sounds crazy, but think about it. Your body is this amazing, complex machine that is always trying to tell you a story about how it is doing, whether it's good or bad. A symptom is a story the body is trying to tell. For example, if your child has eczema, the body is telling a story that the skin is inflamed and toxins are trying to get out, which then causes a rash and alerts you there is something out of balance. Does the skin need a cream that will drive the eczema in deeper, or is there something that the child is eating that is an irritant and causing a rash, or is there an imbalance in the bacteria of the digestive system? These are the questions we need to be asking rather than trying to just relieve symptoms.

A great example of this is a little two-year-old boy named Wyatt. Wyatt was assigned to me because he had behavioral issues caused by possible sensory processing problems. After meeting Wyatt and his mother, I found out that he was born with eczema from head to toe, had twelve different food allergies, and his mother was on antibiotics throughout the entire pregnancy due to a liver problem she was experiencing. His mother said Wyatt was moody, did not sleep, and hated to be dressed or bathed. After looking at him, I couldn't blame him. Wyatt had open, weeping sores from head to toe. He appeared to be in pain with every movement he made. I realized then that he did not have a sensory problem; he had a "gut" problem. I explained to his mother that he probably did not have enough "good" bacteria in his digestive system, but rather had too much of the "bad" bacteria. This was causing food to leak into his bloodstream, which in turn caused his entire body to be inflamed. The eczema was a way the body was trying to push the toxins out. Wyatt started on a probiotic to help balance out the "gut" with good bacteria. When I came back two weeks later, his mother reported he was happier, sleeping through the night, and bathing became so much better. After four weeks, his eczema was almost gone. He was retested for food allergies, which decreased from twelve to only three allergies. His mother reported that she had no idea she had been so stressed, until the stress went away and she had a happy, playful toddler.

This is why I am so passionate about what I do. Could it be as simple as if you eat healthy food and take care of your body emotionally, physically, and spiritually then your body will perform naturally to its potential? You bet. My 83-year-old mother is a prime example. My mother is on no medications, is active, feels great most of the time, and always tells me how frustrated she is with all of her friends who are so sick, but will not listen to her. Was she always this healthy? No. In fact, she has only felt this good in the past five years after she quit smoking, drinking, and eating processed foods. Her transformation has been amazing to experience, and I tell her all the time how she keeps getting better. Even at 78 years old, the body can heal itself.

On the other hand, if we eat bad foods, abuse our body with toxins, and are emotionally and spiritually depleted, then our body will (over time) become ill. Symptoms are a good thing, because they are the body's way of trying to get your attention to say, "you've pushed me too far and I'm out of balance." Symptoms, can be compared to the warning light that goes on in your car when something is wrong. Patterns of symptoms make up what we call disease and are a response that the body is adapting its function to survive. In other words, "we rob Peter to pay Paul," if you're old enough like me to remember this phrase. This means the body will rob nutrients from one part of the body to compensate for another part of the body that isn't getting what it needs. If we continue this pattern over time, our body starts to break down and the disease process will take over. Our society has come to believe that we are a "victim" of our body and that we have no control over what symptoms or disease we have. We blame heredity and bad luck on what illness we might manifest. Heredity does play a role in what markers of a disease we might have, but it is up to us to what extent we push the body out of balance as to whether we manifest a disease or not. Your genes do not dictate whether you get sick or not. **We are responsible for our own health**. We live and die at the cellular level, and we cannot be healthy if our cells are living in a sick environment. The food and the lifestyle we fuel our body with today, dictates how healthy we will be in the following years.

So, the next time your child gets another ear infection and the doctor recommends antibiotics for the tenth time, are you going to think, "ear infections run in my family" or could you ask, "is there possibly something causing the ear infections that I should look at?" Remember, symptoms are the clues or the warning light telling us what is out of balance in the body. This is why I am so passionate about starting our kids out with a good nutritional base so as they navigate this crazy toxic world, they have the foundation to fight off disease and live up to their potential.

Germs – Good Guys or Bad Guys?

Kids are messy. They touch everything in sight, especially when they are little. They are one giant GERM carrier, infecting everyone they come in contact with. Is this true or false? Are germs the problem? Is this the reason our children are so sick? I used to think this was the case, until I learned about this amazing thing called the immune system.

So what is the immune system? Our immune system is comprised of the thymus gland, tonsils, appendix, and other organs including the digestive system that protect us from outside invaders, such as bacteria and viruses, that attempt to take over so they can live and multiply. The digestive system is lined with protective bacteria or "flora" that keep us protected from these invaders by providing a barrier to the internal world. This is why the digestive system is our first line of defense for the immune system. The digestive system is coated with these protective, healthy bacteria, so that no invaders such as bacteria or viruses can easily get into the bloodstream, and make us sick. I often get the question, "What herb is the best for preventing colds and flu?" No herb is best. A probiotic (good bacteria or flora), which will protect the lining of the gut wall, is the best way to make sure viruses and bacteria do not enter the bloodstream and weaken the rest of the body. I'll be getting into more detail about probiotics later but in general, probiotics are healthy bacteria that live and grow in the body and when there isn't enough of these healthy bacteria then the bad or unhealthy bacteria are left to grow and cause the body to become out of balance. In fact, 70 percent of our immune system resides in our "gut," so building up the gut wall is far more effective than taking an herb to improve immunity.

Have you ever noticed how obsessed our society is with germs? There is antibacterial everything, from hand cleansers to soaps to shampoos. So why with a country obsessed with cleanliness do we have so many sick people? Believe it or not, our obsession to avoid germs has actually caused us to get sick more. Sounds crazy, but the truth is our immune system wants to work. In order to work, it has to come in contact with everyday common bacteria in order to get stronger. Germs are nothing more than microorganisms. Bacteria or viruses are not responsible for getting us sick, but only look for a suitable "host" to set up house so they can grow and multiply. When the body defenses or immune system are weakened, then germs find it easier to live and grow. However, when our immune system is strong, then it makes it more difficult for these germs to grow because the environment conducive to their growth is not available.

So what causes our immune system to be weakened so that germs can live and thrive? High stress levels, fatigue, poor food quality, lack of movement, and trauma are the big ones. Over time, the body tries to fight back and accommodate. When these factors are continuous, then our 100 trillion cells become weak and germs take over; therefore, we live and die at the cellular level. Such things as trauma are immediate and cause the immune system to take immediate action, whereas allergies or asthma are a result of an overburdened immune system in overdrive now causing symptoms such as inflammation, which then leads to mucous and other symptoms. When this happens, most people will seek out medications for relief of symptoms. This is where the vicious cycle begins. Medications help to relieve the initial symptoms. Over time, medications will compromise the immune system, which often leads to a new set of symptoms that leads to a new medication. Antibiotics are an example of a medication that gets the immune system off track. A typical scenario I see with the kids I work with is a child gets an ear infection and then takes antibiotics. This initially gets rid of the bad bacteria however antibiotics take out both the good and bad bacteria. The ear infection is now gone but the "good," or protective bacteria has been wiped out, leaving the stronger, "bad" bacteria to proliferate and grow. This stronger, "bad" bacteria then causes the breakdown of the gut lining, which leads to a weaker immune system because now the gut lining which was a barrier is broken down and viruses or other unwanted bacteria slip into the bloodstream through this broken down "gut" wall. The child continues to catch more and more viruses because the immune system is now weakened and the germs have now moved in permanently. This, in turn, leads to more antibiotics, and the vicious cycle continues. These kids never seem to get well and often end up with digestive or gut issues due to so many antibiotics, which damage the gut lining and lead to food sensitivities and other health-related issues.

So, am I saying antibiotics are bad and should not be used with treating illness? No, but maybe asking a better question when your child has an ear infection would help prevent this antibiotic roller coaster. Could there be a food intolerance that is causing the ear infection or inflammation in the first place? What about the "good" bacteria that has been stripped away? Maybe there is another strategy that could help with ear infections such as chiropractic care, probiotics, or herbal eardrops to counter the bacteria. At the end of the book, there is a section on specific childhood ailments and a variety of natural strategies are suggested for each issue that can be used instead of only using antibiotics to combat illness.

Could it be a balancing act between building the body up with nutrient dense foods, proper rest, movement, and feelings of well being, while at the same time cleansing the body of toxins that overload the liver and kidneys? I believe it's a balancing act between building and cleansing the body so that the body continually maintains that homeostasis in order to ultimately aid in "healing itself."

CHAPTER 2

The Body Burden – Is Your Bathtub Full?

With more than 80,000 chemicals on the market, it's not surprising that most babies are born with over 400 different chemicals in the umbilical cord blood. These babies are polluted even before they take their first breath. In order for the body to function optimally, it must be able to detoxify or get rid of the constant toxins it comes in contact with every day. So what happens when the toxic load is more than the body can handle? This is known as the "body burden" and happens when the liver and kidneys are so overburdened with an excessive amount of toxins. Instead of getting rid of these unwanted toxins through the elimination organs (i.e., Bowels, urinary tract, lungs, lymph, skin), it has to recirculate the toxins within the body, often compromising the immune system and weakening tissues and organs, causing a person to become sick.

So what is the "body burden"? It basically means, how full is your bathtub with dirty water? What? Visualize this, when we are born we come in with a certain amount of toxins, passed down from our birth mothers, which have accumulated in our organs and tissues. If the mother has a heavy "body burden" or toxic level, from a life time of ongoing stress, and a unhealthy lifestyle, then that is passed down to the child. So let's say the child comes into the world with a bathtub half full of toxins, then he/she has only half the ability to deal with the toxins coming in to his/her own liver and kidneys.

Detoxification and cleansing were not talked about 20 years ago, because this is a natural function of the body. Now, because we are all so full of toxins from our toxic environment, our detoxification organs need extra help just to stay well. Detoxification means improving your body's ability to get rid of toxins and minimizing your exposure to them. Our body is constantly eliminating or detoxifying through our detoxification organs, which include our digestive system, liver, kidneys, skin, lungs, and lymph system. If any one of these channels of elimination is blocked, then toxins build up causing illness or disease.

Elimination – The Cleansing Process

What are these channels of elimination? I learned from my naturopath studies, they are called "The **Bulls**." This stands for: Bowels, Urinary, Lungs, Lymph and Skin. "The **Bulls**" are a primary component of wellness. No matter if you are an infant or 100 years old, they contribute to whether we are well or sick. If your body is unable to get rid of waste from any one of these five systems, poisons back up and the disease process begins. So let's take a closer look at each of these elimination processes.

Bowel – Our bowel or large intestine is our primary organ for eliminating waste. It is part of the digestive system, which is considered to be the "hub of the body" since every toxin comes through this system first. If we do not have a bowel movement one to two times a day, if it isn't formed like a soft banana and if it has an overpowering pungent smell, then we have a channel of elimination that is blocked, causing toxins to build up in the blood. The liver, which is also part of the digestive system, is the body's primary detox organ and is responsible for over 5,000 processes in the body. The liver filters toxins and dumps them into the digestive system to be eliminated. If there are too many toxins for the liver to filter out or if the bowels are not eliminating properly, then toxins will accumulate throughout the body. Many toxins are stored in the organs or tissues of the body, causing chronic inflammation, which is then linked to such illnesses as allergies, asthma, arthritis, and other health issues.

Urinary System – The kidneys are our primary organs for filtering the blood. This filtration system is very complicated, but the end result is excretion of urine. When toxins build up in the urinary system, urine will often be a darker yellow, cloudy, or have a pungent odor. Urine should be clear, look like the color of white wine, and have very little smell. Many people are chronically dehydrated, which is often indicated by the dark color of urine and a pungent smell. These symptoms may be indicative of an infection or the body functioning at an acidic pH (this will be discussed later). Water plays a key role in the detoxification process and is important in keeping the blood clean and kidneys from being overburdened.

Lungs – We often take for granted how amazing the lungs are and that they, too, help with elimination. We breathe in oxygen, and breathe out carbon dioxide. The elimination of carbon dioxide not only keeps us alive, but it helps to keep the blood clean. Often times many of us are breathing very shallow, which compromises this system. Exercise helps to eliminate these gases more effectively. "Diaphragmatic breathing," or deep breathing, helps to bring the body back to a more calm state and helps to manage stress.

Lymph – The lymph system is a network of tissues and organs and is part of our immune system. It consists of nodes, lymph fluid, and vessels, and is responsible for moving lymph fluids throughout the body so that toxins in these fluids can be eliminated. When lymph nodes get blocked, toxins build up and can sometimes lead to cancer because these toxins are not being moved, but are stagnant. There is about 700 lymph nodes in the body and they are located under the arms, groin, and deep in the body around the organs. The tonsils, adenoids, spleen and thymus gland are also part of system and help process these toxins for elimination. The lymph system depends on movement to keep things flowing, and exercise, massage, and jumping on a trampoline are excellent ways to move the lymph.

Skin – Our skin is the largest organ in the body and is also known as the alimentary system. Most people don't think about the skin as being an organ, but this organ can be a huge part of detoxification. Toxins are constantly being eliminated through sweat. It is important to let the skin breath, which means make sure the skin is sweating. I used to be one of those people who did not sweat (even when I exercised) and would often use heavy antiperspirants, which blocked sweating all together. What I did not realize was that by blocking this elimination system, I was contributing to making my blood dirty and adding to my "body burden." That is why it is important to use deodorant instead of antiperspirant because it doesn't block the sweat but just covers up the smell. Make sure the deodorant is as free from toxins as much as possible, meaning no aluminum because aluminum is a heavy metal and toxic to the body. Whatever goes on the skin is absorbed in the body. I often say, "If you will not eat it, then do not put it on your skin."

The Compromised Immune System

So, now we know how the "body burden" contributes to disease and illness by blocking our detoxification process. What about how it impacts the system that is supposed to protect and keep us from getting sick—our immune system? The immune system is very complicated, and its primary function is to protect us from pathogens (i.e., viruses, bacteria, etc.), which can get a hold of a system or organ of the body and cause chronic illness or even death. Our immune system consists of a variety of killer T cells (basophils), which are triggered when it comes in contact with pathogens or cells it does not recognize as healthy. All of the orifices of the body are lined with millions of healthy bacteria which make it more difficult for pathogens to enter and invade the body. These healthy bacteria are also along the lining of the small intestine which provides a barrier that does not allow pathogens to get into the digestive system or for digestive bacteria to get into the bloodstream. This is what I call the "first line of defense," because if the digestive wall is strong, with healthy bacteria, then the immune system has less work to do. Often, autoimmune diseases are a result of the immune system being overburdened and being turned on too much, therefore attacking itself. This often happens when a person has a "leaky gut," where the lining of the small intestine has very little beneficial bacteria, too much bad bacteria, and small holes that allow pathogens to easily slip through into the bloodstream and set off an immune response.

I have noticed, since working as an occupational therapist over the past 30 years, that children are coming into this world weaker and with less ability to fight illness. As I mentioned before, a big reason why I went back to school to become a naturopath, was because of the amount of sick children I was working with who were on so many medications, and not getting any better. I knew there had to be a better way to keep kids well and prevent them from getting sick in the first place. This reminds me of twin boys that were born extremely premature and were struggling with allergies, asthma, and eczema. After learning from their mother that they were on IV antibiotics for over four months, it occurred to me that maybe the reason they could not get any better was because their immune system was overcompensating and that they did not have enough healthy, good bacteria in their gut. I suggested that she start giving the boys probiotics (healthy, beneficial bacteria) and slowly their allergies got better, and they rarely had asthma attacks and didn't need their medication anymore. Occasionally, I will hear from their mother about a skin rash that will creep up. I then will remind her to start up on probiotics again and to avoid food irritants for a month such as foods containing gluten and casein, and sure enough, this helps clear everything up within a week. Besides not having enough beneficial bacteria in the gut, there are many other factors that contribute to compromising the immune system.

Processed Foods

Who does not love fast food and junk food once in a while? The key words are "once in a while." Americans, especially our children, on average eat 70 percent of their food from processed foods. In my work as an OT, I come across many children who struggle with "picky eating" and will often eat only a select few processed foods. These foods often have an addictive quality, and some children won't eat at all if these foods are not offered. When reading labels on many foods, you often will find a long list of ingredients no one can pronounce, as well as additives, coloring or flavorings that do not come close to being real food. These foods will often have **high fructose corn syrup and hydrogenated oils.** Both of these additives are used to intensify the flavor and provide a longer shelf life. The problem is that both of these additives affect the integrity of the cell membrane, making it hard like a candy coated shell along with creating a sticky quality to the membrane so nutrients have difficulty getting into the cell and waste to get out. Why is this important? Remember, we live and die at the cellular level, so this actually contributes to the death of a cell and has been linked to diabetes, hardening of the arteries, and other health issues.

It often can be difficult to navigate the processed food world. In general, follow these simple rules:

(1) Eat foods as close to one ingredient as possible, i.e. banana vs. banana flavored.

(2) When reading labels, look for the least amount of ingredients; do not eat foods you cannot pronounce.

(3) Avoid high fructose corn syrup, hydrogenated oils and foods that contain GMOs (genetically modified organisms).

(4) Avoid food dyes, colorings, flavorings, and any other artificial ingredient.

Pesticides/Herbicides

Picking out fresh foods often becomes difficult because of what is sprayed on fresh produce and the feed given to animals that contain pesticides, antibiotics, and hormones. Whenever possible, buy organic. This is not always easy and can be costly, but the trick is knowing which foods you should buy organic. So, what does it mean to be organic? Organic means food that was produced without using pesticides, antibiotics, herbicides, or fertilizers made from chemical products. This also helps to keep the body burden low, with less toxins to excrete through the detoxification process, leaving the body with more energy for other important bodily processes.

When shopping for fruits and vegetables, you should follow the "dirty dozen" and "clean fifteen" rules. Check the Environmental Working Group's (EWG) dirty dozen list at (ewg.org/foodnews) for more information on pesticides that are in our food. The dirty dozen are the 12 foods you should always buy organic because they are heavily sprayed with pesticides and have thin skin. These include: apples, celery, cherries, tomatoes, cucumbers, grapes, sweet peppers, nectarines, peaches, potatoes, spinach and strawberries. The clean fifteen are foods that have thick skins and generally are not sprayed with pesticides, so they do not always need to be organic. These include: asparagus, avocado, cabbage, cantaloupe, corn, eggplant, grapefruit, kiwi, mango, mushrooms, onions, papaya, peas, and sweet potatoes.

Proteins such as dairy, eggs, meat, poultry, or fish should be organic, wild caught or purchased (whenever possible) from a farmer's market. Often, foods at the farmers market are close to organic because they do not feed their animals feed that contain antibiotics, growth hormones, or pesticides, and they are close to what they should be eating (i.e., grass, worms, bugs, etc.), but they don't always want to go through the expensive process of being certified organic. Often we think that it is more important that our produce be organic rather than our protein source but when you think about it based on the food chain, proteins will be more concentrated with pesticides than produce would be. Therefore, whenever possible opt for only organic protein even if you have to eat less of it because those concentrated pesticides, hormones, antibiotics, and artificial ingredients are more concentrated too and only add to the body burden.

Antibiotics and "GUT" Function

Health care has changed dramatically in the past 50 years, with a focus more on treatment rather than prevention. Health care has made amazing advances, but many of these advances have actually hurt our children more than they have helped them when overused. One of these advances is the use of antibiotics. Antibiotics are amazing at stopping infections, but when they are overused for ailments like ear infections, colds or other minor respiratory problems, this can lead to breaking down the fragile "gut" lining (small and large intestine), leading to a compromised immune system. Antibiotics work by killing bacteria in the body, but unfortunately the protective and beneficial bacteria that live in the "gut" also gets wiped out in the process. These "good" or beneficial bacteria are the body's first line of defense of the immune system for keeping us healthy. When the beneficial bacteria gets wiped out, then the "bad" bacteria are left to proliferate and grow, creating an imbalance of bad bacteria and leading to other "gut" issues such as SIBO (small intestine bacteria overgrowth). SIBO is common in such ailments as Crohn's Disease, Colitis, and Irritable Bowel Disease. The overgrowth of "bad" bacteria often leads to a breakdown in the gut wall, thus allowing food, viruses, and other organisms to slip into the blood stream. The immune system can then go into overdrive and ramp up to make more immune fighting antibodies, leading to constant inflammation. This then leads to autoimmune diseases, food sensitivities, digestive issues, and the person constantly being sick because the protection of beneficial bacteria is wiped out, often leading to more antibiotics. Think about it. Have you ever wondered why there is a gluten-free aisle at the grocery store now, or why so many children have allergies? When "gut" function is broken down, it impacts the function of the rest of the body.

Environmental Toxins, Heavy Metals and GMO's

With the amount of toxins in the environment, our children are up against a losing battle. Children have a smaller body mass, which means their body has limited capacity to detoxify. Our fast, modern lifestyle has led to pesticides, preservatives, heavy metals, and GMOs (genetically modified organisms). These all play a part in making detoxification a difficult process.

Heavy metals are often used in the making of vaccines, along with being in our air and soil from factories. Heavy metals, such as mercury, aluminum, arsenic, and lead can break down the tissues of the brain and nervous system. Mercury is especially dangerous due to its ability to break down the myelin sheath, which is the protective fat coating along our nerves and in our brains. Heavy metals are often difficult to break down and detoxify, so they often get stored in the organs and tissues of the body. This can contribute to chronic issues such as inflammatory diseases, and neurological issues.

GMO's are plants or animals created through the gene splicing techniques of biotechnology. By interfering with the DNA of the species, the idea is to create a product that can withstand any insect or bug, therefore yielding more food. GMOs have been linked to neurological problems and other health issues and are banned in most countries, although still allowed in the United States. According to Melissa Diane Smith who has written a number of books on GMO's and *Going Against the Grain,* "80% of all GMO crops are engineered for herbicide tolerance, which has led to herbicide-resistant "super weeds" and 527 million more pounds of herbicides have been used since GMO crops were introduced in the USA 16 years ago." The long-term effects of GMO's are not well understood, but many researchers believe they have contributed to the increase in food allergies in the past 16 years. Smith also indicates serious health risks with livestock who eat GMO products, including, infertility, organ damage, and cancer. GMO foods include: corn, sugar beets, yellow squash, zucchini, canola, papaya, alfalfa, and soy. If these foods are not labeled Non-GMO or organic, then they are genetically modified. GMOs are also in most processed foods with those ingredients. A few states are seeking legislation to label genetically modified foods more readily so the consumer is more informed.

Vaccines

The subject of vaccines tends to be controversial, with varying opinions in the health world regarding the pros and cons. This is a health freedom, which should be protected and left up to the family and individual whether to vaccinate or not. It is important, wherever you stand on this issue, to do your research so that you can make an informed decision. Complications and symptoms from a vaccine may include: high fever, fatigue, high pitched screaming, irritability, and seizures. Other countries in the world tend to vaccinate much less than the US and start vaccinating between 3-6 months old because the immune and nervous systems are more developed and mature. The controversy over vaccines continues, due to research supporting a correlation between infant mortality rates, along with the increase in autism over the years. In 1970, only 7 vaccines were required in the US and now 49 vaccines are mandated by 6 years of age. In 1975, Japan raised the age to 2years of age before starting to vaccinate and had the best infant mortality rate in the world. In 2002, Japan changed its vaccine schedule and children now receive 6 vaccines in 12 doses by age five and still have the best infant mortality rate. Other research has indicated that it is not the vaccine that is the issue as much as it is the additives in the vaccine, such as aluminum, formaldehyde, adulterated viruses, bacteria, and thimerosal (methylmecury) that may be causing problems. These issues include poor gut integrity, cellular damage especially to the brain due to toxins crossing the blood brain barrier, and other immune and nervous system issues.

If choosing to vaccinate, it is important that the child is healthy and displays no symptoms of illness. Since a vaccine is an insult to the immune system, the immune system should not be compromised when receiving a vaccine. A few days before and after the vaccine, double doses of Vitamin A and C are recommended to boost the immune system. Using essential oils, such as lavender, topically at the injection site can help draw the poisons out and decrease inflammation. Homeopathic Thuja, in capsule form, which is a homeopathic remedy, can be dissolved and placed under the tongue and is helpful to reduce the pain at the injection site. Rescue Remedy, which is a Bach Flower Essence and helps with emotional stress, is helpful to give by mouth, right after the immunization has been given. Receiving only one vaccine at a time can be less of an insult to the immune system, and is why vaccines should be separated and spaced out.

Delaying vaccines is another strategy that is helpful; as previously mentioned most developed countries wait until the child is older before giving the first vaccination. The use of homeopathic nosodes are another strategy for helping children build up an immunity to a disease. A nosode is a homeopathic remedy that works on the same premise of homeopathy in which "like cures like" therefore, like a vaccine there is a nosode for each of the diseases it is trying to prevent. The body builds up antibodies for the specific disease after receiving the nosode dose, which is made from non-toxic disease material and given orally. Nosodes are made at a homeopathic pharmacy and only administered by a Homeopathic Practitioner. Homeopathy is FDA approved and is used in Europe and other countries as the first mode of treating illness. It is important to remember that strengthening the immune system is the most important piece to staying healthy and preventing disease.

CHAPTER 3

Building Your Kid's Tank –
Building Kids Up Naturally

Cleaning Up The Diet

In a time when it is difficult to compete with a meal that includes a fabulous toy, it is no wonder why parents have given up on making nutritious meals and taken the easy way out by purchasing fast food. I was once one of those parents who fell for the convincing advertising and desires of my children. I thought I was feeding my kids healthy meals until one of my kids was diagnosed with Irritable Bowel Syndrome, and the doctors wanted to put her on medication. I knew I had to walk my talk and really change my child's diet to what I knew and believed in my heart. This was one of the best experiences I could have had as a parent. It taught me that this transition to eating healthy is a continuum of slowly making changes, and eventually these small changes turn into habits. I also learned that navigating this food thing is not as complicated as I thought. It was a matter of cleaning out the processed foods and replacing them with foods with higher quality ingredients. Switching my everyday products such as ketchup or peanut butter to higher quality ingredients meant avoiding products with **high fructose corn syrup, hydrogenated oils** or ingredients I could not pronounce to products with just one ingredient. I then threw out any processed food that had any added sugar. After that, I slowly moved to eating more whole foods, which meant cooking more and having snack foods that were as close to one ingredient as possible. Often, on weekends, I would make a large pot of homemade soup, rice and beans, cut-up vegetables and fruit and stopped hearing "mom, there's nothing to eat." In preparation of most of these dishes, I would use healthy fats (coconut or extra virgin olive oils) with lots of organic spices so that these meals would not only be good for us, but tasty and satisfying. During the day, the kids would snack on these foods, and I would make a simple dinner at night, which consisted of a protein (i.e., chicken or fish), fresh-roasted vegetables, and a gluten-free grain of brown rice or quinoa. Over time, this approach of eating a diet mainly consisting of minimally-processed whole foods, along with specific supplements and superfoods, eventually healed my daughter's gut and has been a way of living for all of us.

SUPERFOOD Me

In a world that is more about "Supersizing" rather than Superfoods, it is no wonder our children are so depleted. The average child by the time he or she is 18 years old will be on 4.1 medications. Childhood obesity is growing at an epidemic rate, and this generation of children will be the first to not live longer than their parents.

Obviously, something major is going on with our food system. It is no wonder everyone, including our children, needs extra help.

Does this mean they should be taking supplements? Well, they need to supplement with something to get the nutrients that are missing from the food they're eating. Even organic food does not have all of the nutrients food had 50 years ago due to a number of reasons, but mainly due to the depletion of the top soil layers, which is caused when land has been over processed and depletes the nutrients that are in the soil.

Supplements that are in pill form miss the boat on the goal to give extra nutrients to the body. Most supplements are made in a laboratory where the nutrients are isolated. These supplements are difficult for the body to break down, because the body only knows what it knows and that is to break down food. Often, these types of supplements cannot be broken down and end up excreted in the urine. When shopping for supplements, it is important that the supplement says "whole food" on it, because in this form the body is able to more easily absorb it. If there are digestive issues, a liquid form of a whole food supplement is even easier to break down.

This is where "Superfoods" come in. What is a "Superfood?" It is any food in its whole form that provides a variety of phytonutrients, which is often a complete food that contains, carbohydrates, proteins, and fats and is high in antioxidants. As a Naturopath, I often get asked what my favorite supplements are. I explain that I prefer "superfoods" or herbs, because the nutrients are coming from what the body recognizes, FOOD.

Superfoods for Kids

Healthy Fats – These are often lacking in the diet, therefore, they need to be supplemented. Healthy fats include omega 3 fats such as cod liver oil, flax seeds, chia seeds, and hemp seeds. These fats are important for brain development, decreasing inflammation, and balancing hormones in the body. Since good fats are the body's healing nutrients, it is important to get a variety of fats throughout the day to help heal the membranes of the body. Other healthy fats include expeller pressed coconut and extra virgin olive oils and a variety of nuts and seeds. Dosing depends on the size of the person, but generally one tablespoon of cod liver oil (flavored) per 100 pounds is beneficial.

Probiotics – These are beneficial bacteria in the form of fermented foods or in capsules or powder. These bacteria are important for digestive health and provide a balance of "good" bacteria in the "gut" so that the immune system stays strong. These healthy bacteria can help with regulating a variety of digestive issues such as gas, bloating, constipation, diarrhea, and food sensitivities. An infant should start with at least 3 billion bacteria with one strand, which is usually bifidus, while a toddler should take 5-10 billion bacteria with at least 3-8 different strands or different types of healthy bacteria. An adult dose is generally anywhere between 20-50 billion bacteria and at least 8-12 different strands.

Green Foods – These are any dark green foods and are typically vegetables, sea algae or wheatgrass. The green color indicates that they are high in vitamins and minerals. Wheatgrass alone contains 92 vitamins and minerals. These foods are pure sun energy, which is why they are green from the high level of chlorophyll. Naturally high in antioxidants, these foods help to decrease inflammation and help to build the body up and provide energy. These foods often have a bitter taste, so are difficult to get into children. Juicing greens or wheatgrass and then mixing the juice of these greens with other sweeter fruit juices is often the best way to hide the bitter taste. Incorporating at least one green food a day in your child's diet is a sure way to not only mineralize them but also to help provide the energy needed to be on the go.

The Digestive System – The Hub of the Body

We have all heard of the saying, "You are what you eat." Did you know the digestive system is the "hub of the body?" Every system and tissue in the body is affected by how well the digestive system assimilates (breaks foods down for absorption), and how well it eliminates (releasing toxins from the elimination organs). Therefore, every disease process starts in the "gut." Billions of bacteria line the entire digestive system from the mouth to the anus, and if any part of this system is not working right, it will directly affect the rest of the system. The chemistry of the body, also known as pH (potential of hydrogen), is involved in each stage of digestion, and has a specific pH to support the function of that system.

To understand this further, let's look at each part of the digestive system and how it can impact the rest of the body. Digestion starts in the mouth and requires an acidic pH to help with breaking down food. Chewing your food properly sets the stage for every function of digestion. Chewing activates digestive enzymes (i.e., amylase), which help break food down so that when the food reaches the stomach, the stomach has minimal work to do. The esophagus is the transit tube to the stomach and has an alkaline pH. This alkaline pH makes it easier for the body to produce mucus to help lubricate the food so it passes through the tube more easily. The stomach is a small pouch with a thick mucosal lining and the contents should be very acidic. The acid environment is important because it helps get rid of the pathogens that are trying to catch a ride into the body, along with helping to break down proteins.

Many children are on reflux medications or antacids, which create an alkaline environment in the stomach where it is important that the pH be acidic. This can cause the food not to break down properly, along with making it difficult for nutrients to be absorbed in the small intestine. These types of medications should only be used in extreme cases, because they can interfere with digestion and assimilation. Acid reflux is often not caused by having too much stomach acid, but rather by not having enough. Usually, by eliminating foods that produce acid such as sugar and simple carbohydrates such as gluten and by taking a teaspoon of either apple cider vinegar or lemon juice in water will eliminate these issues. Working with a Naturopath, to take supplements that help build the gut lining, along with taking the proper amount of probiotics, will usually take care of the issue.

Once the stomach finishes its job of breaking down food further and turning the food into chyme, which is a digestive fluid made up of digestive juices and partially digested food, it then is ready to pass into the small intestine. In the small intestine, this is where we assimilate, or take in the nutrients, from our food. It is the area where most digestive issues occur because there isn't enough healthy bacteria lining the small intestine to create that barrier to the rest of the body. This is also the place where many neurotransmitters are made to balance the brain's chemistry. When there are plenty of "good" bacteria in the "gut," it will make many neurotransmitters that are important for balancing brain chemistry and stabilizing mood. In fact, 85 percent of serotonin (the "feel good" chemical or neurotransmitter) is made in the "gut" rather than in the brain. Understanding this concept is important for helping to keep a child happy and balance those brain chemicals.

As an OT, I work with many children with a variety of mental health issues such as ADHD, autism, sensory regulatory issues, anxiety and general fussiness. These children usually have significant "gut" issues and often have a "leaky gut" where small holes in the small intestine allow food particles or viruses to slip into the bloodstream, causing food sensitivities and often leading to chronic inflammation and ongoing health issues. This is why it is so important to have a barrier of good bacteria that lines the small intestine and does not allow anything to slip through.

This connection between the brain and "gut" is very real and is usually the first place I look when children are experiencing fussiness, mood swings, or digestive discomfort. When food reaches the small intestine to get ready to assimilate or take in nutrients, the accessory organs known as the gallbladder, liver, and pancreas assist in this process. The pancreas has the job of helping to neutralize stomach acid, produce digestive enzymes, and regulate blood sugar. The liver, which has over 5000 functions, is involved in digestion by helping to make bile. Bile is an alkaline substance stored in the gallbladder that helps to emulsify fat so that the small intestine can absorb nutrients. This is why, when the gallbladder is taken out, most people end up with diarrhea because very little bile is released to keep the digestive juices alkaline. These juices are then too acidic for the small intestine to absorb, so they end up passing through the body quickly to prevent damage.

The last part of the digestive system is the colon, or large intestine, and it is mainly responsible for elimination. When children are constipated (i.e., hard, dry stool, or slow transit time) or having diarrhea (i.e., stool moving too fast), then toxicity will build up in the body along with poor assimilation of vital vitamins and minerals. This is why it is important to have enough good bacteria in the gut, along with getting enough water and fiber to help with moving the stool along.

Often, when children have damage to this "gut" lining, many health issues arise. As mentioned before this can happen due to a variety of reasons, but more often than not it can be the result of medications. Medications can break down the lining and antibiotics, in particular, wipe out the "good" along with the "bad" bacteria, which strip the "gut" of the healthy, protective bacteria. This starts a vicious cycle of the "bad" bacteria taking over, causing overgrowth of the "bad" bacteria to create poisons that alter brain chemicals and increase inflammation throughout the body. This often leads to food sensitivities, due to food slipping through the digestive lining and floating in the bloodstream and further causing more inflammation.

When food sensitivities occur, is the answer to avoid those foods forever? Initially, it is important for children with both food allergies and sensitivities to avoid the offending foods. A three to six month time frame is often enough time to avoid the offending foods if these foods are just sensitivities and if the person is also working on repairing the "gut" lining. For a true food allergy, it is important to always avoid these foods and carry an "epi" pen to prevent anaphylactic reactions.

Repairing the "gut" lining requires a number of steps. First, it is important to work with a health practitioner or Naturopath who specializes in digestive issues. Taking the correct amount of probiotics is crucial for building up the healthy or "good" intestinal flora, along with other supplements to help repair the lining, such as aloe vera juice or L-glutamine. The use of digestive enzymes can help with the further break down of food and take the burden off the stomach. Supplements to support the digestive system and repair the "gut" include:

Probiotics – At least 1-3 strands (types of different bacteria) and 1-3 billion live bacteria for infants; 3-8 strands and 3-10 billion for toddlers, and 8-12 strands, and 20 billion or more for adults. Found in grocery, drug stores, and health food stores. Comes in powder form, capsule or "gummy" type.

Plant or digestive enzymes – Taken at the beginning of meals to assist the stomach to break down food for easier digestion. Enzymes are catalysts which help to break down food. These enzymes come from plants and is why fruits and vegetables rot so easily. Make sure there is a variety of enzymes including amalase, protease, lipase, cellulose, and bromaline. They are usually in powder form or capsule and can be found at any health food store.

L-Glutamine and Aloe Vera Juice - To help with repairing the lining of the small intestine. L-glutamine is an amino acid used to repair mucosal linings. Aloe Vera is a plant used for its medicinal properties of cooling and healing.

Fiber – Ground flaxseeds, chia seeds, or psyllium hulls mixed in water or juice to help with bowel transit time to "sweep" the colon clean. Only needed if there is not enough fiber coming from the food.

Water – Enough water throughout the day to allow for good transit time in the bowel, but not too much that the digestive juices are diluted, so drink only 3 ounces at mealtime.

pH – Balancing Body Chemistry

So, what is this thing called pH that so many health practitioners talk about? The letters in pH stand for potential of hydrogen, which indicates whether hydrogen ions are either added or subtracted from a food or drink and determines whether the chemical environment of a living species is balanced, acidic or alkaline. We often think about pH when talking about the water in a fish tank or swimming pool. If the water is too acidic, then the fish dies or the water burns our skin and eyes. If the water is too alkaline, then usually there is too much algae and it sets up an environment for bacteria to grow. The key is keeping the pH balanced.

To measure pH, there is a scale that goes from 0-14, one being most acidic and 14 being most alkaline. Food, beverages, thoughts, and emotions have a pH value. For example, stomach acid has a pH value of 1, soda is 2.8, water is neutral, and baking soda is 12. The human body functions most optimally between a pH of 6.8-7.2 and will use mineral reserves in the body to help maintain that balance. The body gets the mineral reserves from foods and beverages that are high in minerals, such as fruits, vegetables, and mineral water. If the body doesn't consistently get minerals from food, then it has to take minerals from the blood, tissues, and bones of the body, making the body overly acidic, and then the body starts breaking down.

pH is measured from either urine or saliva using pH paper. Most fruits, vegetables, prayer, meditation, deep breathing, and positive thoughts have a higher alkaline pH, whereas processed foods, grains, proteins, fats, sugar, negative emotions, and stress have an acidic pH. Does this mean that we want to strive to only eat fruits and vegetables? No, it is about balance. We need protein and fats, so it is important to get at least 30 percent of our foods from good fats and protein and 70 percent from fruits and vegetables. Therefore, a diet that is mostly plant based but has good fats and proteins is the perfect balance. The reason we hear so much about alkaline pH being healthy is because most of us are too acidic. Think about it. Stress, processed foods, coffee, alcohol, sugar, and negative emotions are consuming our everyday life. It makes sense to try to balance pH by adding more alkaline foods, beverages, and activities. The most important piece is balance; if the body is out of balance, then it is difficult for nutrients from food and supplements to be assimilated. The body is always going to find balance. If the body is unable to find balance from what we put into it, it will take from our mineral reserves. In other words, it will take from our body, and start breaking down.

BIG Gulp – Keeping Kids Hydrated

What are our kids drinking? In talking with families over the years, most parents say that getting their kids to drink water is almost impossible. Juice or milk is the drink of choice for most kids. If their kids do drink water, it is usually mixed with juice or some other flavor enhancer and they drink it all day long. This led me to ask the question, why are these kids so thirsty?

I am often asked by my staff to do consults with children who are "picky eaters." What I usually find after doing the food intake interview is that most of these kids would rather drink than eat. They usually drink large quantities of juice or milk all day long. Therefore, they are not hungry for food. Often, after further inquiring, I find it's the sugar in these beverages that keeps them addicted to beverages, and prevents them from eating real food.

As we have become more aware over the years about how unhealthy pop is, parents have replaced pop with just another version of sugar called juice. I am not talking about the kind of juice that you fresh squeeze from fruit, but the kind that is purchased from the store.

Children naturally have an affinity for sweet foods and drinks, so that is why it is so easy for kids to get hooked on juice.

Water should be the drink of choice for children. Our bodies are made up of 75 percent water; we require water to stay alive. If we do not get water from our food or drink, our body will rob water from or bowels and blood causing us to become fatigued and constipated. Water is required for detoxification. When we are dehydrated, we are more likely to become sick because our body is overloaded with toxins that it is unable to get rid of.

The easiest way to get kids to drink water is to offer it from the very beginning. I made this mistake with my children. My first born son was hooked on watered-down juice. By my third child, I offered her water only. To this day, she prefers water and my son prefers sweetened drinks. There are a few simple ways to make water taste better: infuse water with fresh-cut fruit, put in a few drops of citrus essential oils, such as lemon or orange, or put in a few drops of a natural sweetener called stevia, which often comes in different flavors. Stevia comes in a liquid form, making it easy to add a few drops to water to give it a slightly sweeter taste. This will make water taste better, but will not be so sweet that it overwhelms the taste buds like flavor enhancers or sweetened drinks can.

How much water should our children be drinking, and does it matter what type of water they drink? In general, we should all be drinking half of our weight in ounces. For children it is more important to limit the sweetened drinks and offer water as their beverage of choice. Children usually, when it is offered to them, will drink the amount of water that is right for their body. Sending a large water bottle to school with them will help them stay hydrated and alert. Types of water such as tap vs. spring water are important. If your child is drinking tap water, make sure there is a filter on the tap to remove toxins and especially to remove chlorine. Chlorine is very damaging and disrupts the delicate balance of the "good" bacteria in the "gut." If your child is drinking bottled water, then spring water is best because it contains minerals. Mineral water is especially good because as the name says, it has minerals in it. It usually is in a carbonated form and a fresh squeezed juice can be added as a special treat that is very alkalizing to the body. Drinking at mealtime, primarily, should be avoided because it dilutes digestive enzymes. Up to three ounces with meals will not be a problem, since most children need liquid to aid in swallowing of food. Drinking liquids should primarily be done between meals.

CHAPTER 4

The Natural First Aide Kit

As consumers of traditional modern medicine, we have experienced the side effects that accompany conventional medicine. Children, because of their small body mass, experience those side effects more than adults, so it is important to keep their body burden low by using as many natural remedies as possible. This can be done by creating a natural first aid kit that is created from ingredients in your kitchen, along with herbs, homeopathy, essential oils, and Bach Flower Essences. For the past eight years, I have been using mostly natural remedies for minor ailments such as colds, flu, headaches, skin issues, and digestive issues with my family.

Essential Oils

Essential Oils or aromatherapy are man's first medicine and date back as far as 2000 years ago. These oils have been used by physicians, priests and by a variety of cultures, with 188 references in the Bible alone. They are aromatic oils distilled from plants, which make them 100 times more concentrated than dried herbs and flowers. Essential

Oils are used to stimulate immune health, kill bacteria and viruses, detoxify and help balance the emotions. These oils contain oxygen molecules, which make them powerful and are more easily carried into the cells of the body while being gentle enough for babies. Every living creature has a bio-electrical frequency expressed as hertz (Hz). Plants have a frequency of 0-15 Hz, herbs have a frequency of 15-27Hz, and a healthy body has a frequency between 62 to 78 Hz. Processed foods are considered dead food, therefore they have a Hz value of 0. Essential oils have a frequency of 52-320Hz, making them the most powerful remedies for healing the mind, body, and spirit. Children especially respond well to essential oils due to their small body mass so the oxygenating molecules have less area to cover. They tend to work quickly but gently because of their oxygenating effect, and they are safe for infants and toddlers but working with a Naturopath or Aromatherapist is advised for exact dosing.

How to use Essential Oils

1. **Topical Use** - Most essential oils tend to work best when delivered through the skin. They need to be diluted with carrier oil such as almond, jojoba or a favorite pure massage oil. Dilute the oils more for children than for adults, with a ratio of 8 drops of essential oil to a 4 ounce carrier oil. These oils can then be applied to the bottom of the feet, since there are large pores on the feet, making essential oils more easily absorbable. They also can be applied in the general area where there is an issue, such as on the stomach area for issues with digestion. A reflexology chart of the feet is an excellent way to deliver oils to specific areas of the body, because each spot on

the bottom of the feet corresponds to a specific organ or area in the body. Reflexology points of the hand are not a place for essential oils because of the likeliness that they might get into the eyes or face.

2. **Inhalation** - Use a diffuser or a steam inhaler to ease respiratory distress or to bring the therapeutic benefits of the oil into the air. Use for short periods of time, about five to ten minutes.

3. Always carry essential oils in glass bottles, and store in a cool, dark place. Essential oils can damage plastic.

4. Children generally should not take essential oils internally, unless it is a citrus oil such as orange, lime, grapefruit, or lemon and only one to two drops.

5. If experiencing any irritation or reaction, discontinue use and remove with coconut oil.

6. **DIY Cleaning Products** – Make your own cleaning products to keep children safe from harmful chemicals. Add essential oils of lemon, lavender or any other favorite oil to distilled water to make a spray cleaner or to a washcloth to make a dryer sheet.

Favorite Essential Oils for Children

1. *Lavender Oil* – Universal oil and can be used for most anything; induces sleep and relaxation, calming, balances emotions, relieve headaches; diffuse or topical application to bottom of feet

2. *Lemon, Orange, or Citrus Oils* – Uplifting to the psyche, cleansing, great to make into cleaning products or to diffuse in air to balance emotions

3. *Oregano or Thieves Oil* (Young Living Company) – Anti-viral, anti-bacterial; prevent colds and flu by applying to bottom of feet

4. *Peppermint Oil* – headaches, nausea, digestive issues; applied to back of ear or diffuse

5. *Eucalyptus, or RC Oil* (Young Living Company) – Respiratory issues, asthma; applied to chest area or diffused in air

6. *Peace and Calming* (Young Living Company) – Anxiety, stress, insomnia, great with hyperactive children; applied to bottom of feet

Bach Flower Essences

Bach Flower Essences work to address emotional well-being through the use of human energy fields. Very similar to homeopathic remedies, these remedies are made from the bio-magnetic energies of flowers and plants. Bach Flower Essences were developed in the 1930s by Dr. Edward Bach, who was a physician and homeopath who researched how the energy patterns from flowers have a very specific bio-magnetic energy that influences patterns of emotions. Like homeopathic remedies, flower essences are highly diluted and made into a tincture by distilling flowers in water at the peak of their flowering. Bach's research found that when the mind is experiencing stress, there is often an impact on the physical body causing the body to have a lower disease resistance.

How Flower Essences Work

Bach was one of the first healers to realize that emotional balance strengthens the body's ability to resist disease, and these flower essences help to assist that balance. Each flower has a specific vibrational frequency that matches a specific emotional frequency. Therefore, the impatiens flower helps to balance a person who is feeling impatient. Since these remedies are so diluted, they are very subtle and gentle and, therefore, can be used with all ages, including children and pets. The remedies most often come in a liquid form that is made into a tincture, and a few drops are placed under the tongue. They also can be delivered in a spray, cream, or pastilles, which are small candies to suck on. There are 38 individual remedies that correspond to a specific emotion that is out of balance, along with combination remedies for stress and sleep. The most common **Bach Flower** remedy is a combination of five flowers called **Rescue Remedy** and is used for feelings of stress and anxiety. This is a must have, and I always carry it with me for any situation where there is emotional upset. Bach Flower Essences can be found in most health stores in the homeopathic section.

How to Make and Use Bach Flowers

Bach Flower Essences are sensitive to vibration, as are homeopathic remedies. Therefore, the tip of the dropper should not be handled or touched, because it can absorb an individual's frequency or vibrational energy. It is also important to keep it away from cell phones, computers, X-ray machines or any other electro-magnetic equipment, because it cancels out frequency. Use a clean, one ounce amber colored bottle and fill it with the remedy (about 2-4 drops), and then fill it up to the neck of the bottle with vinegar. If making a spray bottle, then 15 drops mixed with distilled water is used. Usually, these remedies use brandy as a preservative; when dealing with children, vinegar works just as well. Only six remedies can be mixed in one bottle at a time, and Rescue Remedy can be counted as one remedy. Once mixed, shake vigorously in a vertical manner to help energize the remedy, and do this every time before use. The remedy can then be placed directly under the tongue (4 drops), diluted in water or food, sprayed in the mouth, rubbed on the inside of wrists, or diffused in the air. Use the remedy 4-8 times a day, or more, if the situation is more acute. Use the flower essence that best matches the "out of balance emotion."

The 38 Bach Flower Remedies

Agrimony – Hide behind a cheerful façade and do not want to burden others with their troubles

Aspen – Those who experience vague fears and anxieties for unknown reasons

Beech – Critical of others, find fault with others or things

Centaury – Cannot say "no" to others, desire to please others, and/or easily taken advantage of by others

Cerato – Lack confidence in their own decisions and constantly seek out advice from others

Cherry Plum – Fear of losing control, may have impulses to do things known to be wrong

Chestnut Bud – Those who fail to learn from experiences and repeat the same patterns over and over

Chicory – Those who overly care for others or need to control others, tend to be "martyr" type

Clematis – Those who are spacey, daydreamers, and lack concentration

Crab Apple – Have a poor self-image, feel unattractive, feel unclean, feel shameful from something they've done or has been done to them

Elm – Feeling overwhelmed by responsibilities

Gentain – Easily discouraged by setbacks, wanting to give up easily, doubts abilities

Gorse – Feeling hopeless and despair

Heather – Seek companionship of others who will listen and engage in constant talking

Holly – Overcome by negative emotions such as envy, jealousy, anger, revenge

Honeysuckle – For those dwelling in the past; often homesick or nostalgic

Hornbeam – Not being able to face the day, usually once they get going is able to push through

Impatiens – Those quick to thought or action, very impatient

Larch – Feel inferior, lack self-confidence, and often do not make an effort to succeed

Mimulus – Fears of known things like heights, the dark, etc.; often timid and shy

Mustard – Feelings of deep gloom, which comes on for no known reason and then lifts just as suddenly

Oak – Tend to never give up, those who are over-responsible even during hardships

Olive – For mental and physical exhaustion

Pine – Often blame themselves for mistakes of others, feel they should do better, apologetic

Red Chestnut – Overly concerned for the welfare of others, always thinking bad will happen to loved one

Rock Rose – Experiencing states of terror, panic, nightmares, or easily excited

Rock Water – Those strict with themselves, tend to be rigid in thoughts and lifestyle

Scleranthus – Those unable to decide between two things

Star of Bethlehem – For trauma caused by a loss or sustaining an injury to self or loved one

Sweet Chestnut – Those who feel they have reached their limits of despair-anguish is unbearable

Vervain – Those who have strong opinions, overbearing, argumentative, always need to be "right"

Vine – Those who are strong-willed leaders, always in charge, can be dictatorial

Walnut – Protects against influences when going through any type of change

Water Violet – Those who are independent, aloof, do not interfere with affairs of others, prefer to deal with issues on their own; use to assist with grieving process

White Chestnut – For constant and persistent thoughts that go over and over in your head

Wild Oat – Feelings of dissatisfaction from not succeeding in "one" career or life, unfulfilled ambition

Wild Rose – Feelings of no passion, no fun, resigned self to accept their life circumstances without complaint

Willow – Those who have suffered circumstances they feel were unfair and often become bitter toward life and tend to blame others for their misfortune

Homeopathy

Homeopathy is one of the oldest systems of medicine, developed in the 1800s by Dr. Samuel Hahnermann. Dr. Hahnermann discovered that disease is an energy imbalance and that symptoms are the body's way of telling us that something is out of balance. Homeopathy is based on the principle called **The Law of Similars:** expressed as **"like cures like."** This means that the body has its own "vital force." When given homeopathic remedies that work with the natural laws of healing, the body can heal itself by using these remedies to assist with the healing. This healing is done by matching the very specific symptoms to specific homeopathic remedies to help the body increase its own ability to fight off disease. For example, **apis** is a homeopathic remedy that is made from bees and is used to help with bee stings and insect bites. Unlike conventional medicine, more is not better when it comes to homeopathic medicine. Small amounts over a period of time are more effective, and doses are often given more frequently initially. Then the remedy is discontinued when the symptoms start to get better, indicating that the body is starting to take over and come back in balance. A variety of doses are available and range from 6X, 6C, 9X, 9C, 30X, 30C, 100C, with the lower numbers used for more acute, physical issues and the higher number doses for chronic issues that usually have an emotional component.

There are many homeopathic combination remedies that address specific issues such as allergies, sleep, colic, teething, etc. Boiron and Hyland are some of the most well-known brands. Homeopathy is unlike conventional medicine because conventional medicines try to suppress symptoms, while homeopathic remedies act as catalysts for the immune system to go after the root cause, rather than trying to mask symptoms. Homeopathic remedies can be found in health food stores or pharmacies and are widely used in Europe.

Favorite Homeopathic Remedies for Children

Aconite – Symptoms come on suddenly, intense pain, restlessness, anxiety, fear, often first stages of a cold

Arnica – Usually from trauma such as a strain or sprain, muscle aches, swelling, bruising, and inflammation

Apis – For bug bits or bee stings

Belladonna – Sudden onset of fever, earache, sore throat, often has flushed red face, teething, colds and flu

Chamomilla – Irritable, colic, earache, teething, worst at night

Aconite, Belladonna, and Chamomilla are called the ABC's of Childhood, because they can usually help with most childhood problems.

Gelsemium – Lethargic, cold/flu where there is no energy

Hepar Sulphuris – Colds with constant discharge, rattling cough

Ipecac – Nausea, vomiting

Hypericum – For nerve pain especially in fingers and toes

Magnesium Phosphorica – For abdominal cramping

Mercurius – For diarrhea, greenish discharge with colds

Nux Vomica – Burping, indigestion

Pulsatilla – Asthma, allergies, earaches, indigestion, insomnia

Rhus Tox – Poison ivy remedy and skin rashes

Thuja – Treats warts, moles, and sinusitis

Herbs

Herbal medicines have been used for thousands of years. Most often, people think of herbs as natural drugs, when really they are foods derived from plants with medicinal qualities and can take the place of nutritional supplements. They are used to normalize, balance, and support the cause of the problem, rather than suppress symptoms. This may take longer because herbs work with the body rather than against the body as so many drugs do. When healing with herbs, it usually takes one month of healing for every one year you have had the problem.

A child's body responds well to herbal remedies, although it can be difficult to get herbs into them because of the taste. They usually only need subtle, body strengthening herbs and homeopathic remedies such as teas, syrups, and herbal drops. Herbal dosage for children is done according to body weight. Usually, 1/4-dose for children two to six years and 1/8-dose for infants and babies.

An amazing herbalist named Steven Horne developed the ABC approach, which stands for Activate, Build, and Cleanse. The herbs that activate help to keep the energies of the body moving. The herbs that build help to build the body for strength through nutrition. The herbs that cleanse help to eliminate toxins. Knowing which type of herb (activating, building or cleansing) to use can be tricky, but there are a few easy rules that apply.

Activating herbs help the body to finish the healing process and are usually given at the first sign of illness or symptoms. These herbs tend to be aromatic, spicy or heat provoking herbs. Children usually need more subtle herbs such as peppermint, cinnamon, lemon grass, spearmint, ginger, and chamomile.

Building herbs help to prevent the body from becoming ill and are essential for keeping kids well. Herbs that are building are the immune stimulating herbs. These herbs include: Echinacea, licorice root, garlic, Pau d'arco, Astragulus, Oregon Grape, and elderberry. An herbal vitamin, which is food based, will provide all the minerals needed to help keep kids built up all year long.

Cleansing herbs are the herbs that help to facilitate the cleansing process. Our bodies are constantly in a state of either building or cleansing. The cleansing herbs help to get rid of the toxins in the body so that the body burden is lessened and the toxins can be eliminated. This means opening up the channels of elimination through the bowels, kidneys, skin, and respiratory system. The bowels will eliminate through vomiting, nausea, or diarrhea. Eliminating through the skin might be rashes, hives, itching, or body odor. When eliminating through the respiratory system, the child may have a runny nose, cough, sore throat, sneezing, congestion, or ear aches. The urinary system eliminates with more frequent urinating, back aches, and leg cramps.

Often, we try to suppress symptoms when the goal should be to help the body do what it is supposed to do, which is to eliminate the toxins that are causing the problem in the first place. Children and animals have good instincts about not adding to the body burden and will often stop eating because the body needs a break from digestion. Providing lots of fluids and eliminating protein and processed foods will help to move the illness along faster. Enemas, herbal laxatives, sweat baths, and blood purifiers are just some of the ways herbs can be used to cleanse the body of illness. Once a channel of elimination is opened, the child will typically bounce back very quickly. This is often seen when children are constipated; once the bowels are cleared, they go from being lethargic and feverish to energetic and happy again.

Favorite Herbs for Children

Activators – These herbs help to move things along in the body and are used usually during the acute stage of illness. *My* favorite brands include: Herbs for Kids, Nature's Sunshine products, and Limited Edition Herbs.

- Elderberry – Can be found in a tea or syrup and should be given at the first sign of illness or fever
- Peppermint – Tastes good to children and can be used to settle digestive issues
- Chamomile – Settles stomach and calms nerves
- Yarrow – Bitter herb that when combined with peppermint works well, use for fevers and colds

Builders – These herbs help to build up the body by supplying many trace minerals. *My* favorite brands include: Herbs for Kids and Nature's Sunshine products.

- Echinacea – Supports the immune system
- Licorice Root – Helps to support the adrenal glands, which helps with balancing stress
- Astragulus and Elderberry – Immune fighting herb, anti-viral
- Trace Minerals – Needed in small quantities, but when delivered in an herbal formula work synergistically with the body

Cleansers – These herbs help to cleanse the body of toxins. *My* favorite brands include: Herbs for Kids, Nature's Sunshine products, and Limited Edition Herbs.

- Flaxseed, Blue Vervain, Cherry Juice, Prune Juice, and Licorice Root – Help to move the bowels

- Catnip and Fennel – For digestive issues such as gas, stomachaches, and nausea
- Epsom Salt Baths – Helps to draw toxins from the skin
- Sarsaparilla, Dandelion, and Oregon Grape – Blood purifiers to help cleanse the lymph and kidneys

PART TWO

Health Conditions of
Babies & Toddlers

A.D.H.D./A.D.D.

What is it? ADD (Attention Deficit Disorder) and ADHD (Attention Deficit Hyperactive Disorder) are rarely diagnosed under the age of three but can affect all ages, including adults. There are many characteristics, such as the need to be in constant motion, difficulty attending, impulsivity, emotional problems, anxiety, and difficulty processing sensory information. The causes of ADHD vary, but many children are sensitive to the toxins in the environment and the preservatives in processed foods. The Feingold diet has been highly researched and focuses on eliminating sugars, preservatives, and food dyes.

Remedies to Help

- Elimination Diet – Eliminate gut irritating foods such as dairy, soy, and gluten.
- Avoid processed foods with dyes, preservatives, and added sugar.
- Healthy Fats – The brain is made up of mostly fat, therefore healthy fats such as Omega 3 fats help support the brain. These include flaxseed, Fish oil, chia seeds, and walnuts.

- Whole food diet – Eat mostly foods that are at their original source such as fruits, vegetables, lean proteins, and fats.
- Supplements – Liquid B complex and magnesium help to calm the brain and nervous system.
- Probiotics – Establishing healthy bacteria in the gut is key to brain health.
- Calming herbs – Chamomile and lemon balm are great mild teas for calming.
- Essential oils – Diffuse in a room or put a few drops on a pillow case of lavender, peace & calming, and valor (Young Living Oils).
- Homeopathic Calm Forte (Hyland brand) – This helps with sleep issues.
- Auditory Integrative Therapy (AIT) – Auditory training can help integrate and process different sound frequencies, which can impact the vestibular system to help with regulation.
- Craniosacral Therapy (CST) – Gentle manipulation on cranial and sacral bones can balance cerebral spinal fluid.

ALLERGIES

What is it? Allergies are a reaction in the body such as a runny nose, congestion, headache, fatigue, itchy eyes, and sneezing. There are many things that can cause this hyper reaction such as animal dander, grass, mold, and pollens. In young children allergies are usually related to foods, so it is important to rule that out first. However, as the child gets older allergies can be more related to things in the environment.

Remedies to Help

- Eliminate possible trigger foods such as dairy and wheat. These foods often cause more mucus in the body.
- Supplement with cod liver oil to help reduce inflammation in the body.
- Vitamin C – We burn through our vitamin C more quickly when the body is stressed, so double or triple the dose of Vitamin C.
- Herbs such as astragalus will help to strengthen the immune system and should be given one week on and then a week off during allergy season.

- Strengthen the adrenal glands, which are responsible for producing or stress hormones. Licorice root tea or tincture is helpful on an ongoing basis.

- Use a netty pot with a saline solution to help clear the sinuses and prevent further infection.

- Homeopathic remedies for specific allergy symptoms can be very helpful in managing symptoms. Remember, with homeopathy try to match the symptom as much as possible to find the correct remedy. Combination remedies are made for all allergy symptoms.

- Use an air purifier with a HEPA filter. Diffusing lemon essential oil will help to purify the air.

- Keep the bowels moving since constipation can impact the lungs and keep toxins circulating throughout the body.

ASTHMA

What is it? Asthma is an inflammatory respiratory disease that causes breathing difficulties. The airway swells and constricts, making it difficult for air to get in and out of the lungs. Wheezing and shortness of breath are typical symptoms. Asthma can be triggered by allergies, upper respiratory illness, stress, exercise, and food sensitivities.

Remedies to Help

- If needed, go to the hospital and give inhaled bronchodilator medication to open the airway.
- If having an attack, give one dose of homeopathic **aconite** and a dose of **rescue remedy** to help calm the child and reduce stress.
- Air ionizer or hepa filter help to purify the air.
- Diffuse essential oils of RC or Raven (Young Living Oils) to clear the air of viruses, bacteria, etc., or rub these oils diluted on the throat or chest area.
- Eat a diet of whole foods. Eliminate processed foods that contain dyes and preservatives.

- Eliminate dairy and wheat products, which are inflammatory and create mucus.
- Supplement with Magnesium, two doses a day.
- Supplement with Vitamin C. Dose according to age of child.
- Supplement with Omega 3 fats to decrease inflammation.
- Supplement with a whole food vitamin that has a good amount of B vitamins. This helps to prevent attacks by building the adrenal glands.
- Other adaptogenic herbs (herbs that balance stress hormones) to consider are astragulus, and di-glycerized licorice root (DGL) to increase lung strength.
- Make sure the bowels are moving regularly to help keep the balance of good bacteria in the bowels, which will rid the lungs of bacteria too.

BEDWETTING

What is it? This is also called enuresis, is typically more common in boys than girls, and is not due to bad behavior. Usually it is an indication of a small or immature bladder, emotional stresses, urinary tract infection, or food sensitivities. Full bladder control may not happen until 5-6 years. Bedwetting can be an indication of diabetes, so the child should be tested if prolonged.

Remedies to Help

- Always look at possible food sensitivities. Try an elimination diet of one or more of the following foods: milk, dairy products, wheat, citrus, or sugar.
- Avoid pop, sugary drinks, tea, or caffeine.
- Give liquid magnesium/calcium supplement to balance fluid levels in the body.
- Provide homeopathic remedy, 6x, 9x, or 30c, of cantharis.
- Do bladder stretching exercises, such as holding urine for longer periods of time during the day or in midstream.
- Receive acupuncture or acupressure on the bladder points.

COLDS & FLU

What is it? These are common viral infections that affect the upper respiratory system. Symptoms include: runny or stuffy nose, coughing, sore throat, sneezing, headache, loss of appetite, and achy joints. Flu symptoms typically come on more suddenly, whereas colds come on gradually. When children get reoccurring colds, this is a sign that their immune system is compromised and needs to be uplifted.

Remedies to Help

- Increase intake of Vitamin C at the first sign of a cold and take until bowels become loose.
- Zinc lozenges also fight the infection.
- Avoid sugar because it reduces white blood count.
- REST, REST, REST. Let the child sleep as much as possible to rejuvenate the body.
- Elderberry syrup helps to reduce colds and prevents them.
- Echinacea is an herb that helps boost the immune system and is found in many herbal cold formulas.

- Colloidal Silver is a watery looking substance that is taken by mouth for viruses/bacterial infections. For children, one teaspoon a few times a day works well.
- Thieves essential oil (Young Living Oils) is an anti-viral & anti-bacterial oil to diffuse in air and rub on bottom of feet.

COLIC

What is it? Colic is long persistent crying that doesn't respond to any type of consoling. It is usually related to digestive problems and can be caused by: milk allergy, spasms of colon, immature digestive or nervous system, sensory processing issues, and temperament.

Remedies to Help

- If breastfeeding, watch what the mother is eating such as dairy, caffeine, citrus foods, chocolate, and gassy raw vegetables.
- Switch to a pre-digested formula, lactose-free formula, or goat milk/fresh carrot juice.
- Add probiotics. Lactobacillus bifidus adds friendly bacteria back into the digestive system to balance it out. Follow dosing according to specific brand, found on the back of bottle. Always buy at health food store.
- Homeopathic remedies – Some options are homeopathic colocynthus, chamomilla, any homeopathic blend made by Hyland's or Borion, and Hylands COLIC tabs.

- Infant massage – Massage tummy from below the belly button in a clockwise manner, or in an upside down "U" stroke. Use almond or apricot oil with essential oil of lavender mixed in.
- Sensory processing issues - Swaddle tightly to provide deep pressure touch, pat firmly on bottom or back, vertical rocking (moving baby in an up and down manner), classical music or nature sounds, low lighting, and diffusing essential oil of lavender in the air.

CONSTIPATION

What is it? Being constipated includes difficulty passing stools and pain with bowel movements. Most children should have at least one bowel movement a day (infants have several). Often constipated children will stop eating, vomit, be uncomfortable, or experience pain when passing a stool. Insufficient fluids, food sensitivities, lack of fiber, and imbalance of healthy bacteria in the gut can cause it.

Remedies to Help

- Increase the amount of fluids in the child's diet, such as water, diluted juices, teas, and hot soups. Make sure water is mainly given throughout day and not at meals to avoid diluting digestive juices.
- Whole fruit – Toddlers need at least one piece of fruit a day for fiber.
- Warm liquids or hot cereal in the morning helps stimulate the digestive system.
- Provide foods high in magnesium (the relaxing mineral) such as prunes, figs, or a t of black strap molasses.

- Probiotics – Lactobacillus bifidus is a probiotic that provides friendly bacteria to the gut helps balance out the intestinal flora. Follow directions on back of bottle, and buy at health food store.

- Provide mucilagenus foods that provide a lubricating effect such as ground flaxseed mixed with yogurt, or applesauce. After age 2, give one teaspoon of flavored cod liver oil (Carlsons or Nordic Naturals brand).

- Food sensitivities – Eliminate dairy products, since they are very difficult to break down. Wheat products can also be constipating, and watch that the child isn't eating too many processed foods.

- Give an epsom salt bath (magnesium sulfate), which is the relaxing mineral for the body. Put 1-2 cups in a warm bath.

- Give a tummy massage in a clockwise direction using a natural oil such as almond or apricot oil.

- Drink food grade aloe vera juice or licorice tea. Mix 1 tablespoon mixed with fruit juice once a day.

- Enemas – Make sure they are made of natural ingredients and are gentle enough.

- Go to the bathroom with feet propped up to help with eliminating in a squatted position (i.e. Squatty potty).

CRADLE CAP

What is it? Cradle cap is an inflammatory skin disease that occurs on the scalp of infants, usually in the first months of life, and can be found on parts of the face and groin. Overactive sebaceous or oil glands most often cause it, and it is only a concern if it gets infected. The rash tends to look thick and scaly, and it most often doesn't itch.

Remedies to Help

- Add Probiotics. Lactobacillus bifidus adds friendly bacteria back into the digestive system to balance it out. Follow dosing according to specific brand. Always buy from a health food store for quality control. This helps prevent infection. Also, if nursing, the mother should take the probiotics.
- Rub the scalp with calendula gel or cream.
- Use homeopathic Sulphur, dose 6x, 9x, or 30c, twice daily to counteract symptoms.

CUTS AND BRUISES

What is it? Whenever there is a break in the skin, this is considered a cut. A bruise is when there is a black and blue mark on the skin from injury where the blood vessels have leaked out blood under the skin. Both are typical injuries in childhood, however, they are important to attend to since a small child's immune system isn't fully developed.

Remedies to Help

- Ice and compression can help with swelling when there is a bruise.
- **Arnica Montana** is a homeopathic remedy that can be taken orally, along with rubbing the cream on the bruise to help with inflammation and reduce swelling. Do not apply this remedy if the skin is broken.
- Vitamin C helps with inflammation and healing.
- Apply calendula cream to cuts, as it has an anti-bacterial component to promote healing.
- Bach Flower Rescue Remedy given under the tongue helps with emotional upset.

DIAPER RASH

What is it? This is a rash or inflammation of the skin in the diaper area, usually caused by an acidic reaction of the urine or feces on the skin. Often plastic pants or too tight of diapers trap heat and make the rash worse. An overgrowth of candida albicans (fungal infection) in the digestive system can often cause a rash, too.

Remedies to Help

- Keep the diaper area clean, and wash the area with a baking soda paste to pull out the toxins and balance the acidity.
- Let air and indirect sunlight get to the area for at least 20 minutes a day.
- If a health professional indicates it's a fungal rash, such as candida albicans, then give a probiotic.
- It can often be related to new foods in the diet that are making the feces acidic. An elimination diet of the possible offending food may be helpful.

- A plant enzyme given with food can help break down the proteins in the foods, which make the feces acidic.
- Calendula cream or gel is gentle for soothing irritated skin (Natural anti-septic cream).

DIARRHEA

What is it? Diarrhea is loose, watery stools that usually occur often. Most cases of diarrhea are the body's natural way of getting rid of toxins from a virus or bacteria, and often the child is fine after a day. Hospitalization is needed if the diarrhea is causing blood in the stool, cramping, or dehydration for over 48 hours.

Remedies to Help

- Make sure the child gets plenty of fluids to prevent dehydration.
- Avoid dairy products, fats, and proteins, which are harder to digest. Clear liquids are best, such as broths and coconut water.
- Give probiotics to help balance the good bacteria in the digestive system.
- Homepathic remedies, such as **Arsenicum album** in a 6, 9, or 30x dose, are the most common remedy for diarrhea. Match homeopathic remedies that match the symptoms.
- Essential oils (Di-Gize of Young Living Oils) rubbed on the abdomen area can help with cramping.

EAR INFECTIONS

What is it? Otitis Media is an infection of the middle ear. The Eustachian tube is located in the middle ear, and in most children this tube may be horizontal, making it difficult for the secretions to run out of the tube. When the fluid is blocked or sits in this tube, infection often occurs. As a child grows, the tube curves downward, allowing the fluids to drain better. That's why most children outgrow ear infections.

Remedies to Help

- Antibiotics are often the first treatment, however, they are often overused, lead to digestive issues, and don't address the cause of the fluid.
- Eliminate dairy products, especially cow's milk. These foods often thicken the secretions and cause inflammation in the ear canal, making it difficult for fluid to drain.
- Lactobacillus bifidus is a probiotic that provides friendly bacteria and balances out the bad bacteria.
- Vitamin C is an anti-inflammatory and prevents infections.

- Zinc lozenges or in tincture form helps to boost the immune system.
- Garlic oil/mullein oil drops in the ear will kill the infection and decrease the inflammation. These drops can be found in the health food store and are very effective.
- Chiropractic and craniosacral work often prevents ear infections from reoccurring.

ECZEMA

What is it? Eczema is an inflammatory skin disorder characterized by red, dry patches of skin that can be moist and oozing. This condition can affect any part of the body but is often found in the creases of the body or on the face. Eczema is often associated with food sensitivities or contact dermatitis.

Remedies to Help

- MSM Cream or Calendula Cream helps with itching and pain.
- Spirulina or Blue-green algae powder can be mixed into smoothies to help mineralize body for healing.
- A probiotics provides good bacteria in the gut to help keep the blood clean, which is a direct reflection of the skin.
- A bath with epsom salt and baking soda will pull out the toxins while decreasing the inflammation.
- Omega 3 fats help with preventing and healing skin issues. Cod liver oil (flavored) or flaxseed are best.

EMOTIONAL STRESS

What is it? When a child displays such behaviors as anger, fear, sadness, and withdrawal, it is an indication that the child might be having issues of emotional stress. Children often are unable to verbalize what they are feeling, so it is important to validate the emotion they are expressing and to comfort them. Children thrive when their home environment is consistent and predictable, with clear guidelines to help them feel safe and secure.

Remedies to Help

- Limit processed foods, especially foods containing sugar, which irritate their nervous system.
- Sensory processing issues – Rule out if the child is overstimulated or irritated from a sensation in their environment. Deep pressure touch, such as a firm hug, can help with calming. See an Occupational Therapist if you suspect sensory processing issues.
- Herbal teas such as chamomile or oat straw tea help to calm the nervous system.

– Rescue Remedy is a homeopathic 5 flower essence that helps calm the nervous system and relieve stress. It comes in a tincture form, spray, or pastilles to place in the child's mouth. See the Bach Flower Essences section for a more specific flower essence when addressing a specific emotion.

– Teach your child deep belly breathing to help get the nervous system back into a calm, relaxed state.

– Diffuse essential oils of orange, bergamot, or other citrus oils to help lift emotional energy and bring a feeling of happiness.

FOOD INTOLERANCES/SENSITIVITIES

What is it? Food intolerances usually occur over time because the body is reacting to a food substance that has slipped through the gut wall and into the bloodstream, causing the body to react by making antibodies to the food substance. This is not a true allergy, which is an IgE or immune response causing an immediate reaction such as hives or respiratory issues. Food sensitivities are usually a delayed response and are not life threatening like true food allergies can be. These reactions cannot be detected by a blood or skin test and can only be known by eliminating the food and then reintroducing the food to see if there are symptoms. This reaction is often referred to as "Leaky Gut Syndrome" and is usually due to the gut flora or bacteria being out of balance, causing an overgrowth of the bad bacteria and break down of the gut lining, thus allowing undigested particles of food to slip through into the bloodstream. Symptoms can be both physical and emotional since these antigens bind to receptors in the brain.

Remedies to Help

- Take out suspected food for 4-6 weeks, then add them back in to see if symptoms come back. (Start with dairy products then wheat).

- Take a digestive food enzyme with all meals to help break down food better. These can be found in health food stores as plant enzymes in both powder and capsule form.

- A probiotic helps to repair the gut lining and replace the healthy good bacteria.

- Take an omega 3 supplement such as cod liver oil (flavored) or ground flaxseed to help with inflammation and repair the gut wall.

- L-Glutamine is a supplement that helps repair the gut wall.

GERD (Gastric Esophageal Reflux Disease)

What is it? This occurs when stomach acid leaks back into the esophagus causing spitting up, pain, and erosion of the esophagus. Many factors contribute to causing GERD such as diet, medications, over eating, and enzyme deficiency. Antacids and reflux medications often mask the symptoms and interfere with nutrient absorption.

Remedies to Help

- Avoid foods that increase stomach acid such as dairy foods, wheat, processed foods, sugar, and soda.
- Change formulas to pre-digested, lactose free, or goat's milk mixed with fresh carrot juice.
- Eat smaller meals more frequently to prevent over feeding.
- A probiotic provides good bacteria to balance bacteria in the gut.
- Sit up at least 45 degrees after eating to let gravity help.
- Take a digestive enzyme with meals to help break down the proteins in the formula or food.

- Herbs such as slippery elm, licorice root, and marshmallow are very gentle but effective in healing the gut lining.
- Rub essential oil of ginger, anise, or fennel on the tummy to ease discomfort.
- Massage or body work can be effective in bringing the stomach down and preventing it from pushing up into the esophagus.

IMMUNIZATION RELATED REACTIONS

What is it? Many factors contribute to a vaccine or immunization reaction or injury. The most common reactions tend to be a low grade fever, fussiness, lethargy, and soreness at the injection site. More serious reactions may be seizures, high fever, neurological issues, or even death. Whether to vaccinate or not tends to be a controversial issue with many opinions on both sides. (See section on Vaccines)

Remedies to Help

- **Always** make sure the child is healthy before considering to vaccinate.
- Consider a delayed vaccine schedule in which vaccines start at a later age when the immune system is fully developed (i.e. 2 years)
- Consider giving only one vaccine at a time instead of clustering vaccines together.
- Give Vitamin C. Double the daily dose a few days prior to and after the vaccination.
- Homeopathic Thuja – A 30c dose should be given immediately after injection to help with pain at injection site.

- Essential Oil – Lavender and Purification (Young Living) applied on the injection site to draw out toxins.
- Bach Flower Rescue Remedy – A few drops under the tongue at the time of the injection can help with the emotional stress.
- Probiotics – Maintain a daily routine of probiotics to help increase the healthy bacteria, boost the immune system, and flush out the toxins after the injection.

INSECT BITES/STINGS

What is it? These are minor bites that cause an itchy welt on the body with mild inflammation. Most bites, unless poisonous, can be treated with household remedies.

Remedies to Help

- Homeopathic Apis Mellifica, a 6x, 9x, or 30x dose, will decrease swelling and pain/itching.
- Apply cold compresses or ice to reduce swelling and histamine reaction.
- Make a paste of baking soda to draw out the toxins, or apply apple cider vinegar.
- Aloe vera gel, calendula cream, or Echinacea tincture can be applied to sooth the area.
- If your child develops a respiratory reaction such as wheezing after being stung, immediately go to the emergency room.
- Essential oils of lavender and citronella help to repel insects.
- Garlic taken orally also prevents children from getting bit.

SELF-REGULATION/
SENSORY PROCESSING

What is it? Babies are born with the ability to self-soothe or self-regulate to keep their nervous system in a calm state. They do this by getting feedback from the environment through all of their senses by touch, pressure, sight, sound, sucking, and movement. This requires help from the caretaker to help meet those needs as their nervous system develops. Premature infants have an immature nervous system therefore often have difficulty with self-regulation.

Remedies to Help

- Allow the baby to suck on a pacifier or breast.
- Swaddle frequently throughout the day.
- Use natural lighting or soft lighting.
- Minimize TV use and play classical or soothing music.
- Diffuse calming essential oils such as lavender.
- Vertical rocking or swinging often throughout the day.
- Pressure touch such as massage frequently throughout day.

- Wear your baby in a soft or lycra type sling.
- Limit over stimulation of sounds, lighting, and people, and watch for cues such as crying.
- Use a sleep sack to provide deep pressure input for calming.

SLEEP PROBLEMS

What is it? Sleep issues can be difficulty falling asleep or staying asleep. Problems can occur due to medical issues such as ear infections, reflux, poor nutrition, or sleep apnea. Sensory processing issues due to a poor ability to self regulate, so the brain stays in a constant state of arousal, can also affect sleep.

Remedies to Help

–   Digestive issues – Check for food sensitivities that are causing the nervous system to be in a state of arousal.
–   Multi-vitamin - A food based vitamin taken daily helps to maintain proper minerals to balance and feed the brain.
–   Diffuse essential oil of lavender in their bedroom to help with relaxation.
–   Provide deep pressure touch to the skin by sleeping in a sleep sack or pajamas that snug to provide the calming deep pressure touch.
–   Homeopathic calm forte given before bed is very helpful with calming down the nervous system.

- Adequate movement and exercise during the day is important for helping the brain to calm down.
- Bathing in Epsom salts with lavender oil provides the relaxing mineral magnesium.
- Providing a dark room is key for stimulating melatonin.
- Keeping electronics at least 8 feet away from the child's head is key for eliminating electromagnetic field toxins.
- Taking melatonin an hour before bed may help to induce sleep.
- Vibrating the crib or gentle rocking and swinging before bed can help calm the nervous system.

TEETHING

What is it? Teething includes pain and irritability when teeth are cutting through the gums. Many children become feverish, stop eating, stop sleeping, and have looser bowels.

Remedies to Help

- Homeopathic arnica montana will help with the pain. Homeopathic teething remedy is also helpful.
- Provide a cold washcloth to chew on.
- Amber necklaces found online or in a baby store reduce inflammation and provide relief from pain.

THRUSH

What is it? Thrush is a fungal infection of the mouth caused by the bacteria candida albicans. Symptoms typically occur on the tongue and inside the cheeks, displaying white, flaky, thick patches, and can interfere with feeding. Usually thrush is seen in infants and indicates that the good, healthy bacteria is out of balance throughout the body.

Remedies to Help

- Anti-fungal medications can be helpful, however, it is important to balance out the good bacteria with probiotics once the round of medication has been taken. Follow the dosing on the bottle indicated by the weight of your child.
- Soothe the inside of the mouth by wiping coconut oil or aloe vera gel on the gums and cheeks.
- Treat the mother as well if breast-feeding. She should avoid eating sugary foods or drinks.
- A nursing mother can drink pau d'arco tea to help kill the yeast inside her.

RESOURCES AND FURTHER READING

This book provides a basic start to the how, why, and what babies and toddlers need when raising children using a holistic approach. As stated before, this information is not to replace the advice of a medical doctor but is only intended to empower and educate. All of topics were only touched upon so the following resources will provide a deeper understanding to natural health organizations, agencies, modalities, and products.

HOLISTIC PRACTITIONERS

American Association of Naturopathic Physicians
www.naturopathic.org

National Center for Homeopathy
www.homeopathic.org

American Association of Acupuncture and Oriental Medicine
www.aaaomonline.org

American Holistic Medical Association
www.holisticmedicine.org

International Chiropractic Pediatric Association
www.icpa4kids.com

International Association of Infant Massage
www.iaim-us.com

BOOKS

The Baby Book: Everything You Need to Know About Your Baby from Birth to Age Two by William Sears, M.D. & Martha Sears, R.D. (Little, Brown, 2003).

What Your Doctor May Not Tell You About Children's Vaccinations by Stephanie Cave, M.D., F.A.A.E.P. with Deborah Mitchell

The Unhealthy Truth by Robyn O'Brien (Crown Publishing Group, 2009)

Smart Medicine for a Healthier Child by Janet Zand, N.D., Robert Rountree, M.D., Rachel Walton, MSN, CRNP (Penguin Group, 2004)

Healthy Healing by Linda Page, Ph.D., (Healthy Healing, Inc., 2004)

Gut and Psychology Syndrome, by Natasha Campbell-McBride, M.D., (Medinform Publishing, 2010)

Practical Uses and Applications of the Bach Flower Emotional Remedies, Jessica Bear, N.D., (Balancing Essential Press, 1990)

Food Allergy Field Guide, by Theresa Willingham, (Savory Palate, Inc., 2000)

On Target Living, by Chris Johnson, (John Wiley & Sons, Inc., 2013)

Homeopathic Self-Care: The Quick & Easy Guide for the Whole Family, by Robert Ullman, N.D. and Judyth Reichenberg Ullman, N.D., (Three Rivers Press, 1997)

Fell's Official Know-It-All Guide to Health & Wellness, by Dr. M. Ted Morter, Jr. M.A., (Frederick Fell Publishers, Inc., 2000)

The Holistic Baby Guide, by Randall Neustaedter, OMD, (New Harbinger Publications, Inc. 2010)

Reference Guide to Essential Oils, by Connie & Alan Higley, (Abundant Health, 2002)

Gut by Giulia Enders, (Greystone Books, Ltd., 2015)

Homeopathic Medicine At Home, by Maesimund B. Panos, M.D., and Jane Heimlich, (Penguin Putnam, Inc., 1980)

The ABC Herbal, by Steven Horne, (Whitman books, Inc., 1995)

Cure Your Child With Food, by Kelly Dorfman, MS, LND, (Thomas Allen & Son Limited, 2013)

Nutritional Herbology, by Mark Pedersen, (Wendell W. Whitman Co., 1998)

Practical Uses and Applications of the Bach Flower Emotional Remedies, (Jessica Bear, N.D.)

Products

Boiron, www.boiron.com, (800) BLU-TUBE (full line of homeopathic medicines)

Hyland's and Standard Homeopathic Company, www.hylands.com, (800)624-9659 (full line of homeopathic medicines)

Nelson Bach USA Ltd, www.nelsonbach.com/usa.Html, (800)319-9151, Supplier of Rescue Remedy & all other Bach Flower Essences

Carlson Laboratories, Inc., www.carlsonlabs.com, (888) 234-5656 (Fish Oil & Omega 3 supplements)

California Baby, www.californiababy.com, (877) 576-2825 (Organic products for skin, hair, bath, etc.)

Herbs for Kids, www.herbsforkids.com., (800) 648-2704

Natures Sunshine, www.naturessunshine.com

Limited Edition Herbs, www.limitededitionherbs.com, (574) 269-2800

☺

INDEX

P

pesticides 16, 17, 18

pH 11, 27, 28, 31, 32, 33, 98

Probiotic 3, 5, 7, 14, 26, 28, 30, 31, 54, 63, 66, 67, 71, 73, 75, 77, 82, 83, 86, 95

Processed foods 3, 15, 19, 23, 24, 32, 33, 38, 48, 53, 57, 66, 79, 83

R

Rescue Remedy 21, 41, 42, 57, 69, 80, 86, 100

S

Sensory regulation/processing xii, 2, 53, 63, 64, 79, 89, 91

SIBO 18

Skin xiii, 2, 9, 10, 12, 13, 14, 16, 32, 37, 38, 46, 48, 50, 67, 69, 71, 72, 77, 81, 91, 100

Sleep 3, 39, 41, 45, 54, 61, 90, 91, 92

Stevia 34

Superfoods 24, 25

supplements 24, 25, 28, 30, 31, 33, 47, 54, 55, 58, 59, 82, 100

Symptoms xi, xiii, 1, 2, 4, 6, 7, 11, 20, 45, 46, 47, 48, 56, 57, 61, 67, 73, 81, 83, 95

T

Teething 45, 46, 93

Thrush 95

toxins 2, 3, 4, 8, 9, 10, 11, 12, 16, 18, 20, 27, 34, 35, 47, 48, 49, 50, 53, 56, 71, 73, 77, 86, 87, 92

U

Urinary System 11, 48

V

Vaccines 18, 20, 21, 85

vitamins 21, 26, 30, 48, 55, 58, 61, 69, 75, 85, 91

W

water xii, 9, 11, 28, 30, 31, 32, 33, 34, 35, 39, 40, 41, 42, 44, 65, 73

Printed in the United States
By Bookmasters